# ~SALAD

# FOR

# BREAKFAST~

*WHY TEENAGERS AND ADULTS NEED TO EAT*

*SALAD FOR BREAKFAST*

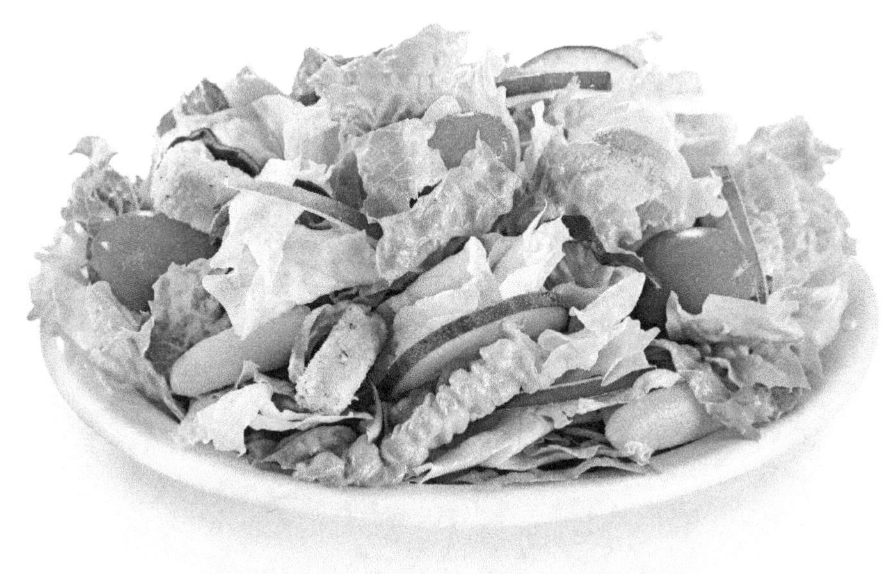

*Ruby Dot Oliver-Hill*

# Table of Contents

# About the Author

Ruby Dot Oliver Hill was born in North, S.C. where she attended high school. Mrs. Dot went to several colleges including, Claflin College in Orangeburg, S. C., Peralta College in Alameda Calif, and Jones Business College, in Jacksonville, Fla. She also received her nursing certification and worked in the nursing field for over 15 years. Prior to being in the nursing field, She worked for many years in banking before retiring from that field.  Mrs. Dot's writing career began a long time ago when she went to Bridgeport Connecticut in 1961. While being there for two weeks, an advertisement came out in the newspaper which said that Norman Rockwell, the cartoonist, needed a writer. In spite of being apprehensive about the position, she wrote a story and then was called in by his secretary who followed up with her for over 6 months in an effort to hire her on as a writer. At that time, Ruby felt that she was too young to do that type of job, even though her younger sister tried so hard to inspire her to go to Rockwell's studio in Norwalk Connecticut.  A couple years after turning down that opportunity, there was a writing contest which was advertised in the newspaper in Washington, D.C.  The article that she submitted about her cat won the writing contest and that article is now featured in the archives gallery. Adding to her list of accomplishments, she is also responsible for creating four inventions. Ruby's life's work has consisted of utilizing her creativity, resourcefulness, and know-how to make a profound impact upon the lives of others, which is what led to the conception of writing "Salad for Breakfast". Lastly, Mrs. Dot is currently pursuing a degree in Public Health and Nutrition, because she is very passionate about people achieving optimal health in their lives!

# *Foreword*

*Many people, especially those specializing in finance, believe that Wealth is our greatest asset, and it is true that without financial resources a person has limited access to material possessions and the limited ability to create independence and stability for themselves. A life lived in poverty is full of frustration, perpetual disappointment, and self-loathing. However, through time and diligence wealth can be attained or replaced if it is lost. But the two commodities of Time and Health are not so easily replaced. The hours of our life cannot be reversed, no matter how hard we try, and the best solution is to go forward and redeem the time by not making the same mistakes and breaking the counterproductive cycle, which we may have established. Although you can regain your health, the aging process of the human anatomy still follows its natural course with or without our permission. Many people are searching high and low in drug stores, vitamin shops, and on the internet for the fountain of youth encapsulated in a bottle or pill, which often doesn't reap the desired benefits. In this insightful and informative manuscript Mrs. Dot, as she is affectionately known, gives us her secret to which has caused her to remain vital and healthy for 80 years! Mrs. Dot has astounded medical professionals during her routine checkups. Even her coworkers have admired her strong work ethic and her ability to perform a strenuous job even into her late 60s and now she wants to share her secret with the world! Pretty soon she will have you eating a salad for breakfast!*

# CHAPTER 1

## *The Necessity of Green Salad for Breakfast*

Regardless of where you live in the world, we all have one thing in common- our health. In order to stay healthy we must eat an assortment of healthy foods such as green vegetables, exercise, engage in yoga, properly handle stress, as well as integrate other key components into our lives. But in my opinion the key ingredient to being healthy is including green vegetables into our diet for an early morning breakfast. This is why I feel so strongly about introducing everyone to try my healthy strategy of eating a salad for breakfast. I have been eating green salad for breakfast for over 15 years every morning. Although there are many different methods to improve your health, I believe that this is a unique, new way for you to become healthy. Come along with me on my journey and listen to the importance of eating green salad for breakfast. I was inspired to write this book from personal experience, because I've witnessed the effects it has had upon my own life. I challenge you to eat green salad just 7 days for breakfast, and see how it will make a great difference in your life!

There are all different types of salad you can eat but green salad is the number one salad for anyone to eat to have a strong healthy body. Let me explain the difference between eating a green salad for breakfast as opposed to eating it for lunch or supper. I have tried eating the salad for dinner after I have worked 8-12 hours (the average person work 8-5 pm and they are tired and worn out after those 8 hours). I realized that I didn't have the necessary energy I needed because I missed out on all of my morning nutrients. However, when I've eaten the salad for breakfast I was ready to go and make a difference whether it was on my job or I was just at home doing chores. If you start your day with a salad you will notice that you are not as lethargic and you don't have to fill up on so many empty calories or fast food. Fast food is another choice that people have for breakfast but that type of food is not very beneficial for the body. Maybe a small amount of the fast food is not as harmful. But you must eat that green salad before you digest all of that non-nutritious cuisine. Just think about the greasy tater tarts, sausage, eggs, and biscuits covered in butter on the top and on the inside. I know it sounds very tempting and mouthwatering as I describe it, but think about how it impacts your body, especially first thing in the morning. Not only the food itself is bad, but many of the places where you currently eat breakfast use a horrifying amount of grease and butter. These eateries say they use oil, but what kind of oil are they using? There are certain kinds of oil and butter that should be used which are healthier for you overall.

You can make your salad any size you desire- small, medium, large, or extra-large. Top your green salad with any fruits, nuts, dried tomatoes, kiwi, walnuts, pecans, almonds, raisins, apples slices, orange slices, avocado or any other type of topping that is healthy.  Make sure you choose the salad dressing that doesn't have a lot of oils in it. Many people make the mistake of going through the trouble of making themselves a very healthy salad but then they top it with the dressing that has the most cholesterol and fat, which is very counterproductive. This is just as bad as preparing a nice, lean grilled or baked chicken and then covering it with a lot of barbecue sauce or ketchup. So stay away from the greasy oils. Of course, I don't personally endorse any one type or brand name of salad dressing and some people may decide to use fat free dressings. You want to capitalize on feeling good first thing in the morning and giving your body a great start with energy and vitality.  Once you start to eat salad for breakfast you can try out a variety of different recipes. I have some great recipes at the end of each chapter but feel free to alter them to suit your individual needs.

Green salad works so well in the early morning because it fills you up. I have found that the best time to eat a bowl of salad is from 6am -9am, during your normal breakfast routine. If anyone wants to lose weight the salad is a very good start for the day and if you drink a glass of water after you eat the salad you will be getting all the necessary nutrients for your body and increasing your ability to burn fat. Taking all those weight loss pills etc. is not as healthy as eating a good source of vitamins and nutrients such as green salad in the morning. If you eat green salad for breakfast you will have a lot of energy, feel good, and look good because your complexion will change and glow. Follow my advice and eat the salad and see what a great positive effect it will have upon your body. With this new boost of energy you will be filled with vitality and strength that you hadn't tapped into before. Your cells and blood will become replenished. Your body consists of billions and trillions of cells and the green salad will supply the vital nutrients for your cells to function the way they are supposed to. The right type of breakfast aids in "low and slow glucose(sugar) release which is believed to keep the energy levels balanced, preventing 'energy dips' as well as providing long satiety between meals, reduce hunger and lower subsequent voluntary food intake. It is argued that  low glycaemic index/load foods are capable of keeping blood glucose levels lower and stable during the course of a whole day, and thus this could be expected to further add to the beneficial effects of breakfast, providing an ideal 'nutritional start' in the morning" (Kamada, 2011).

Remember, our bodies have been exposed to all kinds of air pollution and toxic chemicals from trains, airplanes, tractor trailers, city buses and the list goes on. These toxic chemicals cause the air we breathe in the atmosphere to be contaminated. The sad thing is that this is happening on an everyday basis. That is why it is so important to have the salad breakfast to combat everything that we are exposed throughout the day. Even the water we drink is contaminated.  Therefore, everyone needs the daily green salad to help maintain their pH balance, especially teenagers and adults. pH stands for the potential of hydrogen. A Garden of Life article explains that, "pH levels are designated on a scale of zero to 14, with the lower the pH meaning more acidic and the higher the pH meaning more alkaline.  A healthy range to shoot for pH-wise is between 6.0 and 7.5. The immune, metabolic, enzymatic and restorative processes function better with proper pH levels and the stomach must be acidic so that digestive proteins function properly" (Gemino, 2016). Salad and other nutritious foods impact the body's environment to keep our bodies free of radicals and help our cells to stay healthy and maintain our pH level.  Merriam-Webster defines free radicals as "an especially reactive atom or group of atoms that has one or more unpaired electrons. Especially one that is produced in the body by natural biological processes or introduced from an outside source (such as tobacco smoke, toxins, or pollutants) and that can damage cells, proteins, and DNA by altering their chemical structure" (2019).

Even if you can't win a million dollars in the lottery you

can feel like a million dollars when you switch to this new

diet!

# SALAD RECIPE (1)

8 OZ  CUP MIX  SALAD

1/2 CUP PURPLE CABBAGE (SHREDDED)

2  BROCCOLLI  FLORETS (DICED)

4 SLICE CARROTS (SLICE)

2 KALE FLORETS (DICED)

TOPPED WITH NUTS, RAISINS AND AVACODA

# CHAPTER 2

## *Real Life Application (Proof is in the Pudding!)*

Try the early morning and experience the difference for yourself. All of us are aware of age. As we get older it is much more important to be adamant about staying healthy because the body begins to break down. As you focus on keeping your body fit and strong ask a doctor about taking vitamins also. Many of them will recommend that you eat some vegetables every day. The vegetables used in green salads are raw which is what makes the salad so healthy for you. Cooked vegetables are good, but raw vegetables are priority.

This is a true story just to prove how healthy vegetables such as carrots are for your eyes. I worked with this gentleman and he now lives at a senior facility. He said to me that he eats raw carrots every day and at 93 years of age he sees better than many people much younger than him. He said he had 20/20 vision and that he did not wear eyeglasses and he reads the newspaper every day. He asked "do you know why I have 2020 vision?" and of course I asked him "why?". He went on to explain, "I am 93 years old, I eat carrots every day for my eyes. My mom started me on carrots when I was a boy at 6 years old". I told him I would check with his nurse to confirm because it was so unbelievable! So I checked with his nurse and she confirmed that he was actually 93, has 20/20 vision, and has never worn glasses. She also said that he does in fact eat raw carrots every single day. That was in 2008 when I sat in the facility with him.

This is another true story about the benefits of raw vegetables and salad. I retired from the bank several years ago and I went to work as a CNA in a senior care home. A registered nurse came to me one day and asked "why do you come to work and never complain that you're tired and you always work so fast?" she said it seems like I just kept going and going. At that point she let me know that her and her peers had been watching me so she wanted to know what (vitamins or drugs) I was taking. I told her I wasn't taken anything. She surprisingly said "are you taking some kind of vitamins or steroids or pills? I am serious you got to be taking something! Tell me because I want to take what you are taking." finally I told her that I eat green salad for breakfast and that was my secret. She replied that she had never heard that before. I advised her to try it and she would be walking around at a faster speed like me! A couple weeks later I  asked her had she tried it but she said not yet. I encouraged her that she really needed to try it in order to see how it worked for herself. The entire time that I worked at that facility I did not know I was being watched by my co-workers. However, the nurse and the rest of my coworkers were amazed at the amount of energy and endurance that I had in my 60's!

At one point I had to have surgery on my gums. The nurse took my blood and then afterwards she asked what kinds of minerals did I take? I told her none. She said "your blood is so rich with minerals." I replied to her that I eat green salad and drink Evian water, which she really approved of. After following through with the surgery I had no complications at all. This let me know once again that eating the green salad for breakfast really paid off! Many people eat sweets and too many starchy foods which can cause your body to be susceptible to diabetes and many other ailments. However, salad has the capacity to reverse some of these negative consequences if a person doesn't wait too late to change their lifestyle.

Green salad is good for everyone. Just 2 months ago I was in a grocery store and a lady and I started a conversation about how grocery prices were continuously going up. She said to me "the prices are not going to worry me because I went to the doctor one day when I was not feeling well. He tested my sugar and I had Type II Diabetes." She said she immediately panicked and was in disbelief about what the doctor said to her. He went on to tell her "I will give you medication to take insulin every morning." she said "before you give me any medication what can I do to get rid of diabetes?" and he specifically told her to eat green salad. She followed his orders and now the diabetes is gone (of course she may have made some other changes in her diet as well which aided her in avoiding diabetes). That day I only went in to buy water and realized just by having a conversation how the green salad stopped a woman from becoming an insulin dependent diabetic. This is why I stress the importance of the breakfast salad!

This has not only worked for me, but I just gave you a couple of testimonials of how vegetables and a salad on a daily basis has worked for others. "More than 100 million U.S. adults are now living with diabetes or prediabetes," according to a report released in 2017 by the Centers for Disease Control and Prevention or CDC. The report finds that "as of 2015, 30.3 million Americans – 9.4 percent of the U.S. population –have diabetes. Another 84.1 million have prediabetes, a condition that if not treated often leads to type 2 diabetes within five years" (CDC). So basically millions of Americans can possibly benefit from eating salad for breakfast!

Often times you hear the early morning coffee drinkers, say "I got to have my cup of coffee." Normally, they don't function well without that shot of caffeine every morning. Our bodies very easily adapt to whatever conditions we expose it to. However, if they will turn that coffee into a green salad and have the coffee later then the benefits will be much more rewarding. Some coffee is not good for your body specifically your kidneys. News18 documents that "too much coffee simply means a lot of caffeine, which in turn raises stress levels, can dehydrate your body, can cause problems like heartburn to arise, and the onset of stomach ulcers. All of this caffeine may also increase your heart rate as well as stimulate your central nervous system resulting in a constant headache while elevated adrenaline level and caffeine overdose can lead to hallucinations while sleeping at night or make you jittery" (2018).

This is exactly what prompted me to share this information in a book and help people become aware of how good and healthy green salad is for everyone who has a goal of embracing a healthier lifestyle. It is important to know the facts and get all of the necessary information as it relates to health. Personally, I think that all eateries should sell a good fresh salad for breakfast in the morning. These days many people are very busy getting the kids prepared for school or trying to get to work on time and they don't have time to get up and make their own salad. However, if different restaurants that serve breakfast also served salad in the morning then this may become very profitable for them and result in a win-win situation for their customers. Many restaurants are already providing healthy options for their customers in addition to their regular menu options, therefore salad could easily get added to their menu as another healthy option.

# SALAD RECIPE (2)

8 OZ  CUP SPINACH

1/2 CUP CUCUMBER (DICED)

1/4 CUP CARROT (SHREDDED)

1/2 CUP ROMANIA LETTUCE

1/4 CUP CHEESE (SHREDDED)

3 CHERRY TOMATOES (DICED)

TOP WITH BLUEBERRIES

MANGO (DICED)

NUTS

# CHAPTER 3

## *Eating Salad Should be Priority at an Early Age*

Athletes, both professional and non-professional use a lot of energy to play the different sports that they play on a daily basis. My recommendation is that they start with a green salad in the morning before going out to practice. This will provide a great deal of energy that is required to perform at the high level of intensity in which they do. They will really be fired up and ready to meet any team if they change to this new diet!  Anyone utilizing a lot of energy from the military, teachers, to construction workers, etc. will reap the benefits from the early morning salad. Your daily performance is your key to your success. Eating the green salad is part of that success.

Much like athletes, young people need a lot of energy to stay active and maintain their busy lifestyles. Teenagers are still growing and developing, and they require a healthy diet so that their bodies will continue to grow as it needs to. We must teach the young people at an early age about nutrition and how healthy the breakfast salad is for them. Instead of them eating candy bars and cookies, and snacks that contain so much sugar at an early age they need to be eating salad. Of course, teenagers are attracted to what tastes good so the food they currently eat may taste good it isn't good for their body. They need to be aware of the dangers of the foods that they enjoy consuming and how it will impact their bodies and their overall health. Teenagers are already exposed to information about what foods are good for them but they need an incentive to eat right. At school they have a lot of different sports to participate in. Even when they become college students they are engaged in all types of sports, so it is important for them to build good habits now. If they eat the salad for breakfast their bodies will have a lot of energy, so if the athletes see that then it will help them to make the choice to change to this diet. Even if certain kids are not athletes the most important thing is for them to be mentally prepared for school by eating a balanced breakfast.

The salad helps teenagers' brains function better. While the kids are enrolled in school they're always busy with homework, extracurricular activities or recreational sports. Some school kids are overweight, however if they began to eat the green salad for their breakfast along with some moderate exercise they can lose weight. The salad will make them feel full and they won't crave too much other food afterwards. When they eat the salad I recommend that they also drink a glass of water to refresh the body. As they begin to change their diet to salad in the morning it is possible that this will encourage them to also take on some other new diet changes. I am inclined to focus on the teens and young people at an early age so that they will be mentally and physically fit as they get older.

Unfortunately, a lot of the information in our society today is geared towards adults and the lifestyle changes that they can make. However, the young people of today will become the women and men of tomorrow. So if you start to eat salad at 16 years old and another person starts at 32 who would be the healthiest in the long run? Look at this situation as a competition or experiment and see how within a 16 year period the salad will have improved the overall health and life span of a 16 year old versus a 32 year old:

In 16 years the 16 year old will be 32 years old

In 16 years the 32 year old will be 48 years old

The 16 years old will be healthier because the 32 year old started late

Both of these people actually win because they both receive the benefits of this new diet change. However, the 16 year old will be able to improve their health as their body is still growing instead of waiting until 32 to change their diet, which involves reversing the negative effects of some bad health decisions. This same comparison can be utilized to encourage teenagers to start saving money, which is important also. Although health and life is more important than finances, finances are an intricate part of having a fulfilling life. If a person starts to save $25.00 a month at age 16 and another person starts at age 32 who will have saved the most money by the time they both reach 48? Of course, the 16 year old again because that person started earlier and was wise enough to utilize their time to make a long lasting effect upon their life.

This is why I stress the importance of eating the green salad early in life. Being overweight is not healthy for anyone. Most people eat too many sweets and starchy food fatty foods, which leads to obesity. Unfortunately, obesity is not only found amongst adults, but it is also found in many schools, ranging from elementary to high schools. The CDC found that, "in 2018 the prevalence of obesity was 18.5% and affected about 13.7 million children and adolescents. Obesity prevalence was

13.9% among 2- to 5-year-olds, 18.4% among 6- to 11-year-olds, and 20.6% among 12- to 19-year-olds.  In comparison to adults which is measured at 35.7% among young adults aged 20 to 39 years, 42.8% among middle-aged adults aged 40 to 59 years, and 41.0% among older adults aged 60 and older" (2018).  This early morning salad will help keep anyone and everyone fit and healthy. If the schools were serving salad for breakfast to the children as an additional option it would provide a great avenue to help those overweight and obesity.  Let's help our kids to stay healthy and fit, because they are very important to maintaining the longevity of our society!

My sincere desire is that my book can reach out to teens and young people globally and abroad. It's so very important for the young people to get started at an early age, speaking from experience. The point I am making is to eat your salad early in life as possible so that you can reap the benefits. I have been eating salad for the last 15 years for breakfast, which is what prompted me to write this book, because I saw the benefits in my own life. As a thinker, I always desired to improve my life and I read a lot of information about being healthy. Also, as I became older I became more health conscious and I didn't want to become dependent upon medication to live.

# THE HEALTHY VEGGIE BISCUITS

IF BISCUITS ARE FROZEN BAKE 17 MINUTES

LET COOL 5 MINUTES

CUT IN HALF, FILL WITH SLICED TOMATOES.

PAT DRY

ADD 2 SLICES OF BACON IF DESIRED

CHOP UP 2 TEASPOONS OF ONIONS, BROCOLLI, KALE, AND SPINACH

SAUTE FOR A FEW MINUTES (PAT DRY)

ON THE BISCUIT PUT BACON, TOMATOES, ONIONS AND GREEN VEGGIES.

TOP WITH YOUR FAVORITE CHEESE SLICE

(CHEESE IS OPTIONAL)

STICK IN MICROWAVE OR IN OVEN UNTIL CHEESE MELTS

# CHAPTER 4

## *Helpful Tips*

The other diet change, in addition to salad for breakfast, which I have benefitted from is drinking more water. People should at least drink five to eight ounces glasses per day and if a person is taking medication it is even more important to have the necessary water intake. The New South Wales (NSW) Ministry of Health and the Heart Foundation states "the recommended daily amount of fluids is:

• 5 glasses (1 litre) for 5 to 8 year olds

• 7 glasses (1.5 litres) for 9 to12 year olds

• 8 to 10 glasses (2 litres) for 13+ years " (2019)

As you can see children and teenagers don't need as much water as adults, but they still need it. Eating a green salad and drinking water is just as important as putting gas in your car to go different places. If you don't put gas in your car it's not going any place. Your body is similar to a car, because if you don't eat good green nutrients you won't get to your destination and your body will start to break down also. The salad will get your cells started and the energy will come natural just like when you crank up your car in the morning and the oil begins to circulate through the vehicle. If you can't find time to exercise at least set aside a time just to stretch every day.   Follow the advice of the older gentleman at the nursing facility and eat carrots every day for your eyes. If you're eating carrots on a daily basis all you'll need is 3 or 4 thin slices.

After you eat the early morning salad your body has already started to get your cells upbeat. So after your cells have charged up you'll feel better and be ready to go! after you have made this change in your life and you experience the benefits you will tell your family and friends the sausage, hash browns or tator tots, eggs and bacon are not good for breakfast without the salad coming first. I hope that you won't eat any of those items at all for breakfast anymore, but at least make salad the first thing you eat, which is the point I am making in this book. You know for yourself that each food source has its own individual benefits. Other foods provide their own source of nutrients, although green salad is exceptional.  People who have diabetes and several other ailments should eat salad regularly to achieve the results that were talked about in chapter 2. All of us are aware of one thing; we are getting older every day so we must eat healthy to maintain our body. Fruits, in addition to other vegetables, are very important to eat daily.

So I want everyone today who reads this book to start eating green salad for breakfast. You may decide which to do on a weekly basis: alternate on your salad 3 days, eat a small salad 4 days, eat a larger salad every other day or alternate between a small salad and a large salad every other day. Just make sure you eat green salad every day. Eat your other food as you desire but just make sure you eat the green salad for breakfast. Please don't wait for dinner or supper because you would've have missed out on the boost you get in the morning, as I stated before.

Although you can make it any way you desire to, I have some tips on making the salad.  One great way I like my salad is with shredded cabbage on top of it. Also what I do on a regular basis is to get a large strainer and put the salad in the strainer. Let some cold water run over it for a minute or so to rinse off any harmful particles.  Shake the salad leaves from side to side and then the salad will stand up in the bowl. Try it for yourself and see how the salad reacts to the fresh water. PERFECT!

# THE HEALTHY VEGGIE CROSSIANT

SLICE THE CROSSIANT IN HALF AND USE THE

SAME VEGGIES THE VEGGIE BISCUIT RECIPE

REQUIRES (P. 34)

TOP WITH CHEESE, RAISINS AND SLICED WALNUTS

STICK IN MICROWAVE A FEW MINUTES,

OR UNTIL CHEESE MELTS

# CHAPTER 5

## *Final Thoughts*

Having optimal health is necessary in order to ensure a long satisfying life for all of mankind. Salad and other vegetables are very natural and has been around for many centuries as a part of the diet for humans and animals alike. However, green salad for breakfast is a revolutionary tip for people who are looking to lose weight, become healthier and make an entire life change. In the future the youth will be in control of the society that we are in the process of building for them. Therefore, it is essential that mothers-to-be are adamant about building healthy habits. The baby's cells need some vital nutrients which can be found in the salad. Prenatal care is an important part of the process of bringing a healthy baby into the world and doctors recommend a diet that contains a variety of nutrients from all of the five food groups. Every pregnant woman knows that whatever she eats, drinks or exposes herself to goes directly to her baby.

Many of today's recommended diets or weight-management systems not as accessible as salad. The diets may need to be ordered online, which involve waiting until that specific item is delivered through the mail. However, if you're ready to change your life today and your health is declining from bad eating habits then you can go to the store today and change your life immediately. Immediate results and instant gratification are important in a fast-paced world today. People are accustomed to lightning fast internet, microwaveable meals, and fast food service. Therefore, I personally recommend that you should at least try the breakfast salad before you dismiss it!

In addition to eating salad for breakfast, below you will find some very beneficial tips that are also important to your overall health:

1) Drink water before you take your medication. A half of glass of water is recommended so that your body will absorb the medicine better.

2) Men need to eat tomatoes to help fight off prostate cancer. By the age of 40 men have to start to get the prostate checked but you need to add tomatoes to your diet before you reach this age.

3) Shredded cabbage or coleslaw as well as bell peppers contains a lot of nutrients.

4) Avocados should be eaten regularly because they help keep the arteries clean. Norwegian cod liver oil also has many vital health benefits.

5) The morning salad can be blended into a smoothie for people who don't

normally take the time to eat breakfast.

6) Movement is also key to maintaining vitality, even if you don't participate in rigorous exercise. Do 10-15 minute stretches first thing in the morning and repeat just before going to bed.

7) Poached eggs can be very healthy because all of the nutrients are not boiled out (which is why raw foods, except meat, are good for you). After breaking the shell, drop it in boiling water for 2 minutes. Flip the egg over and let it sit in water for 2 more minutes. Remove from water and season with black pepper, salt, onions, and parsley.

8) Finally, check out the 60 Second Salad Maker. I definitely endorse this for the fastest and easiest way to make your breakfast salad!

# HEALTHY SMOOTHIES

## RECIPE #1

¼ CUP GREEK YOGURT –UNSWEETENED

½ CUP FROZEN BANANAS

½ CUP WATER

½ CUP FROZEN PEACHES

½ CUP FROZEN SPINACH

## RECIPE #2

1 CUP FROZEN RASPBERRIES

½ CUP LOW FAT YOGURT

½ CUP JUICE (ANY TYPE OF LIGHT JUICE

SUCH AS APPLE ETC.)

½ CUP SWATER

***Blend and Enjoy!***

# Works Cited

1. "Coffee Addiction: The Cons of Drinking Too Much Coffee." News18, 29 Jan. 2018, https://www.news18.com/news/indiwo/food-indiwo-coffee-addictionthe-cons-of-drinking-too-much-coffee-1644677.html.

2. "Free Radical." Merriam-Webster, Merriam-Webster, 2019, https://www.merriamwebster.com/dictionary/free radical.

3. Gemino, Marilyn. "PH Balance and Health." Garden of Life, 31 July 2017,

https://www.gardenoflife.com/content/ph-balance-health/.

4. "New CDC Report: More than 100 Million Americans Have Diabetes or Prediabetes." Centers for Disease Control and Prevention, Centers for Disease Control and Prevention, 18 July 2017,

https://www.cdc.gov/media/releases/2017/p0718-diabetes-report.html

5. Kamada, Ikuko, et al. "The Impact of Breakfast in Metabolic and Digestive Health." Gastroenterology and Hepatology from Bed to Bench, Research Institute for Gastroenterology and Liver Diseases, 2011,

https://www.ncbi.nlm.nih.gov/pmc/articles/PMC4017414/.

6. "Adult Obesity Facts." Centers for Disease Control and Prevention, Centers for Disease Control and Prevention, 13 Aug. 2018,

https://www.cdc.gov/obesity/data/adult.html.

7. "Choose Water as a Drink." Healthy Kids, NSW Ministry of Health, NSW Department of Education, 2019,

https://www.healthykids.nsw.gov.au/kidsteens/choose-water-as-a-drink-kids.

# JOURNAL YOUR PROGRESS!

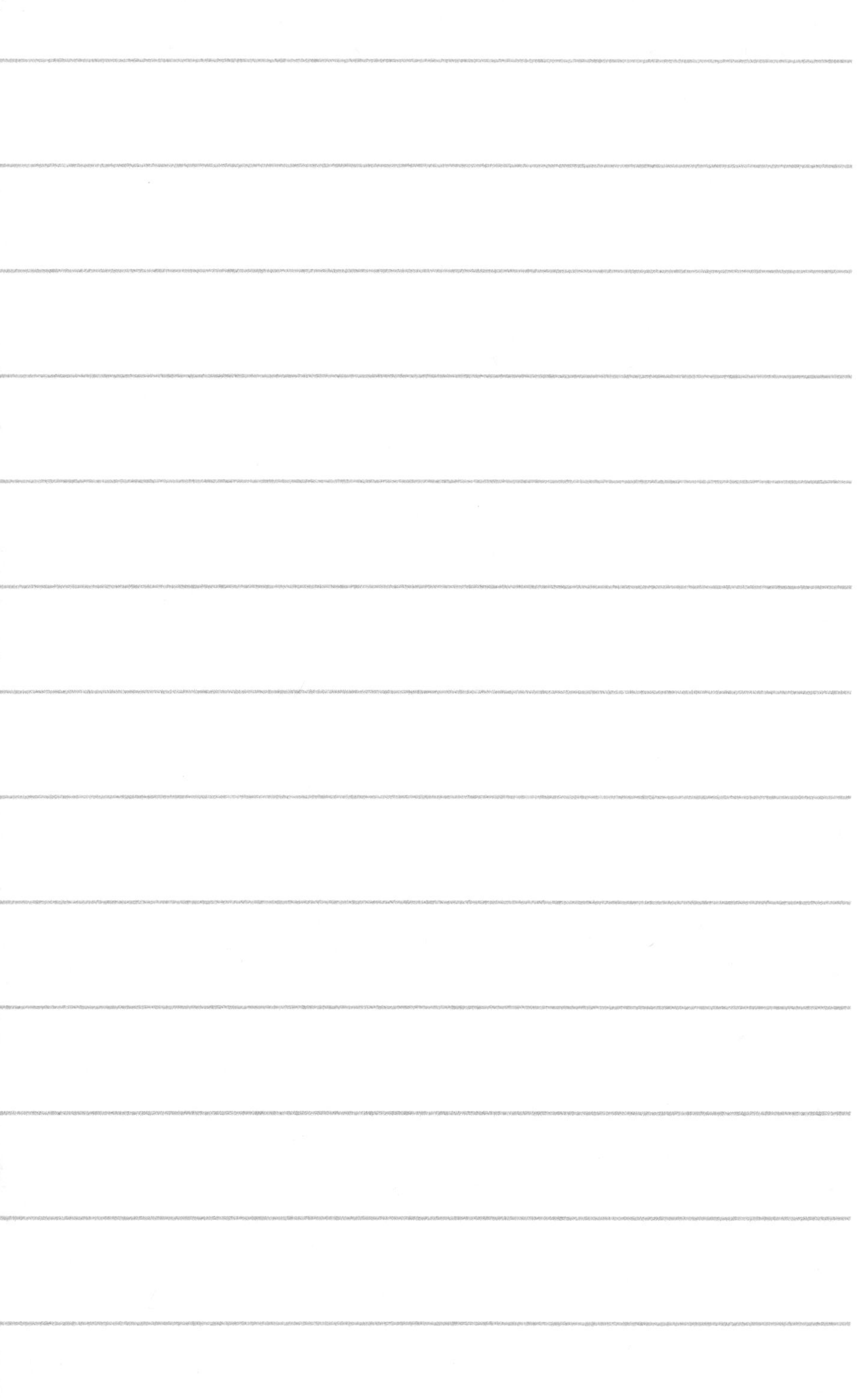